Look Good

365 top-to-to

Kate F.

GW00729235

Smallish Books

SMALLISH BOOKS

8 Clarendon Villas, Widcombe Hill, Bath BA2 6AG

Text copyright © Paul Fisher, 2003

Design copyright © John Brewer, 2003

ISBN 0-9542446-1-3

Printed in China

The guidance in this book is not intended to replace professional medical

advice. Please consult your doctor before altering a health routine.

To:

From:

Date:

LOOK GOOD is a mix-and-match wardrobe of beauty tips that should help you to do what it says on the cover.

The advice comes from talking to friends and family and from my own experience and is therefore the sort of folk wisdom that every woman gathers together. What I've done is to arrange the things I've heard into an informal guide giving various ideas on how to approach everything from hair care to foot maintenance.

Some tips are obvious ("bite lips to redden them . . . wear a G-string to get rid of the visible panty line"); some are new to me ("rub beetroot into the cheeks . . . to remove chewing gum from clothes, put in the freezer and chip off the gum when it has frozen"); some are contradictory ("use a comb with moulded ends . . . I never use a comb"); some strike me as daft ("wear a bra in bed to keep your boobs firm"). All are pieces of individual knowledge that may or may not be useful to you.

LOOK GOOD is a sample of normal women's voices that isn't dressed up as a definitive beauty manual and doesn't need to promote branded products either. It's more gossipy than that; from getting going in the morning to going to bed at night, people know a lot when you ask and I want to thank all those who helped. Especially my Mum.

LOOK GOOD.

Kate Fisher

Laugh at yourself.

I never go to breakfast without putting on my makeup first.

I comb my hair before breakfast and do the rest afterwards.

Beauty is partly an inner thing and if you feel good, you'll look good. So, begin the day with the intention of being nice to others and you can even pay compliments to the grump pots you live with. Occasionally, the compliments get repaid in kind to reinforce the inner you and make the outer you glow that little bit brighter. It won't work every time, but it's not a bad idea.

When I get up I bend over and with my head hanging I pull firmly at my hair until the whole scalp is tingling. It gets the circulation going and really wakes me up.

I keep my slippers by the bed. Why? Because the beautiful woman is a happy woman and the happy woman enters the kitchen with warm feet. And she certainly doesn't ever stub her bare toe on the banisters because she knows that a stubbed toe turns even a goddess into an ugly, screaming heap. That's why I say my slippers are a beauty aid.

Start the day with a good breakfast, and then have three or four smaller meals throughout the day. It will keep you in top form.

First thing in the morning I drink a hot glass of water plus a squeeze of lemon. I do this for the good of my skin and for the good of my soul.

I used to have lots of tips and tricks. Now I'm in my late forties I realise it's more a matter of what you put inside and how you feel. So it's a question of the right foods, exercise and plenty of sleep, cutting back on alcohol, tea and coffee. If you're a smoker, the best tip is to stop. And everybody should drink plenty of water. It's all true.

Consider a new hairstyle. Take your time, study magazines, and consult with the hairdresser. A new hairstyle can be a real confidence booster.

Hair clips and grips used to maintain the same style every day forces your hair into a damaging kind of perm. Vary your daily style regime to avoid this problem.

A quick way to reduce hair static is simply to run your fingers through your hair.

Remember that hot rollers, or any other form of heat styling, runs the risk of brittle hair and split ends.

To check the health of your hair, try the following: put a single strand of hair into lukewarm water; dunk it under the surface and if it bobs to the surface, fine; if the hair sinks, you too will have a sinking feeling because it is time for something to be done to improve your tired locks.

For a treat I mash a banana and massage it into my hair. Then I leave it there until I've repeated – very fast and ten times over – "I mash a banana and massage it into my hair."

To make your hair glossy massage in olive oil, cover with cling film, leave for an hour, clean with a mild shampoo and rinse.

If your hair goes limp during the day, you can give it a boost by tipping your head upside-down, brushing through, then lightly spritzing with hairspray.

Wear a bathing cap at swimming pools to protect the hair from the drying, oil-leaching effects of chlorine.

If your hair goes green after the swimming pool, rub some ketchup into your scalp and then rinse it out.

HAIR care

I use a natural bristle brush because the natural bristle is less damaging on my fine hair. But I think a mixture of natural bristles and nylon gives strength for wet or thick hair.

Paddle brushes with the large flat base are good for long hair.

I use a round brush that has bristles embedded in a metal barrel. This heats up and helps to set and style my hair.

Wash your hairbrush in hot soapy water at regular intervals and pull a comb through it to remove the build up of old hair.

Too much brushing tears the hair and probably pulls it out.

I still go for the old wive's tale (and it's a fair way of describing my mother) of a hundred brush strokes every night to keep your hair shiny. The reason for this is that brushing moves your natural toning moisture from the hair roots to the end of the hair.

Try the one hundred strokes of hair brushing technique with a silk scarf over the brush.

Brush your hair before shampooing to get the tangles out.

Occasionally I do the old-fashioned thing of tipping
talcum powder into greasy hair. It works a treat,
though I wonder whether talcum powder is a beauty
tip or an admission that I'm lazy.

I use a comb with moulded ends . . .

. . . I never use a comb.

Never wash your hair in the bath.

I'm a firm believer that the drier your hair the less it needs washing. When I was in my twenties my hair was more greasy than it is now so I washed it every day. As a forty-something I can now go for two or possibly three days without a shampoo.

You shouldn't confuse lots of lather with clean hair. The amount of lather in a shampoo depends on how much surfactant the manufacturer has included. The same goes for toothpaste and the general rule (which is broken in Australia) is that the richer the society, the more surfactant the soft-soaping multinational will put in the shampoo.

Smooth a tablespoon of castor oil into the hair with your fingers two hours before a shampoo. It makes the hair shine and seals split ends.

I go for a mild shampoo and I set the hairdryer on cold.

I leave shampoo in the hair for at least a minute to fully penetrate the grease. It's the same principle as soaking dirty dishes before you wash them.

To remove excess oiliness, I rinse my hair with distilled water and a splash of lemon juice.

Silly old puritans say hair conditioner doesn't work. They're wrong and should know the glossiest, most shiny conditioners have a pH rating of between 3 and 3.5.

If you want to straighten wavy hair, try to dry it close to the roots, working outwards and brushing each section straight.

My DIY conditioner mixes eight teaspoons of sesame oil with four teaspoons of coconut oil. Heat them up and then add a teaspoon of vinegar and six teaspoons of honey. Work it into the wet hair and then rinse until all the stickiness has gone. It smells great.

Only use a little conditioner on your hair and rinse well.

For greasy hair, use your hairdryer on a cooler setting. A really high temperature will make the scalp produce more oil.

Blow-dry with the nozzle facing down to encourage the split ends to lie flat.

To give your hair a longlasting lift at the crown of
your head, wrap damp hair in velcro rollers,
blow-dry, apply hair spray and then unroll.

Rinse your hair with soda water. The bubbles give
shine and body and the acid base of soda water
helps to thicken the hair.

At the end of a hair wash, spray with freezing cold
water to give a shine.

21

Dry your hair as much as possible with towels before blow-drying to minimise the dehydrating effects of a hair dryer.

When you dry your hair, start by bending forwards for a few moments and letting your hair flop down. This will give it extra height and width.

Brushing wet hair is damaging. You must wait until your hair is dry.

I'm wary of dandruff shampoos and have found they do more harm than good. A gentle comb through is my first dandruff remedy and after that my suggestions are more long term. Try cutting down on starch, fat and sugar, realise stress sometimes plays a part and get out in the sun if you can.

I must occasionally deal with dandruff and do it by adding four tablespoonfuls of dried thyme to a cup of boiling water. I work this cooled and fragrant mix into my scalp after a shower.

I use anti-dandruff shampoo. What else would a girl do?

Eyes are windows on the soul and if you want to alter the glazing, here are a few general makeup tips:

Round eyes: eye shadow should be heavy at the outer corners. Avoid eyeliner underneath the lower lashes and highlight the inner corner of the lid.

Sticky-out eyes: use a dark shadow applied close to the eyelash and blended to a somewhat lighter shade as you work outward. Avoid light and bright colours.

Deep-set eyes: put highlighter on the eyebrows and use two shades of eye shadow with the dark shade applied above the lids and the light shade on the lids.

Small eyes: leave the inner lid paler than the outer lid by blending a dark eye shadow from the centre of the lid. A touch of darker colour above the lashes and applied from the outer part of the lid to the middle also helps.

Close-together eyes: liner and shadow should be taken just beyond the eyes and then blend a lighter shade into the inner corners.

Hooded eyes: shade the entire eyelid and highlight the brow bone with a lighter colour or a bit of fairy dust.

I make my own eye gel to reduce those characterful lines around the eyes. I mix two tablespoons of corn flour with a little rosewater to make a thick paste. Heat in a pan and stir in enough rosewater to make a good consistency. Pour into a small container and allow to cool. Smooth onto eyelids, leave for fifteen minutes and rinse off with tepid water.

25

Everyone should protect their eyes from the sun, the more so if – like me – you have blue eyes. When I buy a new pair of sunglasses, I do two checks. For lens distortion, I hold the glasses as far from my face as I can, then I focus on something slender like a pencil and I move the glasses to and fro. If the pencil appears to wobble, I find another pair of glasses. To test for strength at blocking out the sun's rays, I look at myself in the mirror and if I can see my eyes staring back through the lens, I know they aren't strong enough. Not for my eyes, anyway.

One solution for bags under the eyes is a dab of haemorrhoid cream to reduce swelling.
Go easy with this one, though.

To make eyes appear bigger, put black eyeliner underneath only.

A white line under the eyebrows makes my eyes look more open and bigger.

A spot of lipstick on the inner corner of your eye makes your eyes look brighter.

To reduce bags under your eyes rub a slice of raw potato over the affected areas. This is also soothing on any area of the face.

This is an exercise to get rid of bagginess around the eyes. Lie flat on your back and relax your face then stick your tongue out, pulling it down and extending it over your lower lip as far as possible. Keeping your head still, look up and back, trying to see as far behind your head as you can. Hold it for a few seconds, relax and repeat several times.

To combat fine lines that form around the delicate eye area, circle the index fingers around the eyes. Start at the bridge of the nose and push up and out around the eyebrow, come round under the eyes, but more lightly, and back to the bridge of the nose. Repeat several times.

Before you pluck your eyebrows, soak a flannel in boiling water and dab at the brows at as high a temperature as you can bear. This opens the pores and makes plucking the unwanted hairs far less painful.

Buy really good blunt-edged tweezers.

Pluck your eyebrows only when the moon is waning (getting smaller) as hair grows back more slowly then (supposedly).

If your eyebrows are at all sore after plucking, soothe them with a little tea tree oil.

Brush eyebrows up before plucking to see the baseline.

I put moisturiser on my eyebrows before I pluck them.

To add definition, brush your eyebrows with a touch
of dark brown eye shadow.

A cheap way of highlighting your eyes is to put a dab of
vaseline on the centre of your brow bone.

A little vaseline on the eyebrows helps to keep
them in shape and condition.

Use eyelash curlers before applying mascara.

Invest in eyelash curlers. They make your eyes appear more open and you appear more wide-awake.

Just before you use them, heat eyelash curlers with the hairdryer to make your lashes curlier.

Put a little bit of glistening gold on the eyelids for a party look.

Curl your lashes before lining your eyes or you'll wipe off all your hard work.

A little bit of vaseline separates the lashes and so makes them look longer.

I put vaseline on my eyelashes before putting on mascara.

Put on mascara as two light coats rather than one heavy application that may blob.

Never share mascara because you can spread infections.

Mascara has a limited shelf life of about three months.
After that, it won't do such a good job.

When using eyelash curlers, heat gently with a hair
dryer to seal the curl.

To avoid clumping, leave two minutes
between each coat of mascara.

If your mascara has gone stiff, stand the tube
in a glass of hot water.

When my eyes are really tired, I put white eyeliner on my lower eyelids. This makes my eyes look more open and bright.

Dab a little concealer into the inner corners of your eye sockets to banish darkness.

A damp camomile teabag on each eyelid for ten minutes gets rid of any puffiness . . . I use normal teabags or a slice of cucumber.

For special occasions I use three eye shadows of differing shades from the same group. Working from the inner corner of the eye outwards, I put the darkest shade on the eyelid, the medium shade along the socket line and the lightest shade on the brow bone.

To brighten your eyes without fussing with eye shadow, just run a finger with vaseline on it across your lids. It will give them a natural shine.

Remember that eye shadow usually comes up paler on the skin than in the container because the pigment gets spread out.

If you have close-set eyes, apply a darker shade of eye shadow to the outer third of your eye. If your eyes are wide-set and you want them to appear closer, apply the darker eye shadow to the inner corners of your eyes.

When applying your eyeliner, keep your hands steady by resting your elbows on a flat surface.

When applying eyeliner, try looking down into a handheld mirror.

If you are going out and feeling tired, go easy with the makeup. It will only emphasise the lines.

When you put your makeup on use a really good mirror and have a good light.

If you are using concealer, put it on after the foundation. Otherwise the base just wipes it away.

Only put foundation where it is really needed, such as over broken blood vessels or on uneven skin tone. If you use a compact foundation, put it on with a sponge.

Remember, those with greasy skins need water based foundations without oil while those with dry complexions can kill two birds with one stone and go for a foundation with moisturiser.

Test a foundation on your jaw line and look in the mirror. Trying it on your hand won't be a good guide as your hand is not the same colour as your face. And let the foundation dry before you check.

A darker foundation is no good as a substitute tan. I did it once and looked really weird.

Instead of using powder all over your face, just apply it to the areas most likely to shine, such as the nose and forehead.

For a lighter summer foundation, try mixing a little of your foundation with a blob of moisturiser.

I keep all my makeup and bits in a small toolbox. It keeps the stuff together and looks inviting when I open it up.

If you are going to buy good quality makeup, you should buy good quality tools, brushes and files etc.

MAKEUP

When you are older and applying translucent powder to your face make sure it does not go into any facial lines and make them more noticeable.

When I travel I put my makeup in a zip-up, waterproof, leak-proof bag.

To make makeup last, spray your face with water after you have applied it.

A makeup remover does what it says on the box and no more. It doesn't cleanse the skin of impurities.

I wash my face in plain hot water in the mornings and use a remover applied with cotton wool to take makeup off in the evening. I never use soap.

Soap tends to dry the skin and those with normal to dry complexions should either not use soap or buy a bar of the mildest.

Regardless of skin type, wash with pure olive oil soap no more than twice a day. Rinse face well with lukewarm water.

If you are using a cleanser on your face, leave it on for a couple of minutes so it can really work.

I am suspicious of cleansers and exfoliants and to me it seems more natural to use water for the most part and a mild soap only if I'm really grubby.

Pre-cleanse the skin using cotton wool with liquid paraffin to wipe off makeup and dirt. Actors have used this in the theatre but it's not widely practiced outside and is probably something I shouldn't be recommending to you.

If your skin is looking dull, try a facial scrub to remove dead cells.

When exfoliating your skin, choose a gentle scrub and use gentle motions rather than scrubbing at your face as if it's the kitchen sink.

Exfoliate and scrub your skin more in winter because – with less sun – the speed at which your skin renews itself slows down leaving you more prone to dull, flaky skin.

Simple yoghurt makes a great exfoliating facemask.

My tip for a really good facial is to put tea tree oil into a bowl of boiling water and – a towel over my head – to souse myself in the fumes. I stay under the towel for about ten minutes and keep a kettle handy to top up the water when it stops steaming. Sometimes I finish with a very diluted rinse of sugar and vinegar.

It depends how harsh I want to be on myself, but I like the occasional polenta or sea salt scrub. I flavour it with an essential oil.

Avoid a toner if your skin is at all dry. Many toners contain alcohol or a mild solvent, which may well irritate the skin.

My toning treat is to chill a blend of two parts camomile tea and one part witch hazel.

Mix foundation with vaseline to even out the skin and keep the look dewy.

If I'm feeling skint, I make a toner from rosewater and a few astringent drops of glycerine.

Q: Do you want to know a refreshing face rinse that helps move insoluble residues and restores the skin's pH balance?
A: A tablespoon of lemon juice in a bowl of warm water.

If your skin is oily, post-cleanse with 70 per cent alcohol diluted 1 to 4 parts water. After cleansing with soap, soak cotton wool in the mixture and apply to the skin.

A thin film of liquid paraffin applied to the face and neck at night and in the morning is an efficient moisturiser. It goes on easily and hardly ever irritates the skin. (It conserves moisture by hindering evaporation from the skin.)

I'm not a big one for motherly tips, but I do tell my daughter to go easy on the moisturiser. She has a normal young person's oily skin and doesn't need to know about the dizzying array of moisturisers on sale. That comes later in life.

Keep the room temperature as low as possible. Dry and over-heated rooms take up moisture, so save on fuel bills and your skin.

There is all sorts of nonsense about oval, square, oblong, round and triangular faces. I stopped studying geometry after GCSEs and my definition of face shapes is that everybody is either a bun face, a bird face or a horse face. Check out the mirror and you'll recognise a bird, a bun or a horse staring back at you. I have some hair-styling and makeup rules you might like to follow. Or you might find them nonsense. Anyway, here goes:

Bird faces need a full fringe to emphasise the chin and to narrow the forehead. Highlighting the temples, brow and jaw can have the same effect and birds sometimes benefit from foundation towards the top of the forehead, the cheeks and the chin.

48

Bun faces should stay away from central partings and slim the face with a side parting. An impression of roundness is diminished by long cuts with a short fringe. As for makeup, the bun face might consider highlighting the brow bone and chin and applying a dark shade of foundation to hollow the cheeks out.

Horse faces are big on the jaw and it's as well to keep the hair below the jaw line and avoid well-defined fringes. Straight hair on a horse is often less than flattering so take attention away from a naturally long face by going for a fuller style of cut.

If you have a round or square face, avoid a fringe, as it will emphasise your face shape.

If you have a big nose, use shading down the side to reduce the size.

Keep your face in shape and make the skin feel firmer with the following set of exercises:

* roll your eyes from side to side;
* move your chin from side to side, working all cheek muscles;
* smile broadly and then frown.

Some aren't happy with the shape of their lips and, if so, here are some tips to alter the appearance by more than just a shade of lipstick:

Full lower lips can be hidden with a fractionally lighter shade of lipstick on the top lip than on the bottom lip.

Big lips appear to shrink a bit if you put one of the more mutely coloured outliner inside the actual line of the lip and fill in with a lipstick of the same shade.

Thin lips appear to enlarge with outline applied to outside the lip line and then filling in with a marginally deeper colour.

For softening lips, apply a coat of vaseline and leave for about a minute. Brush off with a toothbrush to remove any dead skin and then apply another thin coating of vaseline.

A lip brush is the best way to do your lips and if at the end of the evening there are some hard-to-shift flecks remove them with sellotape. Just press down gently and peel off.

Pale lipsticks make your lips look fuller, even more so if you put gloss over the top.

After you have put your lipstick on, dab some lip-gloss into the centre of your lower lip. This creates the illusion of all-over lip-gloss but means that it stays put and doesn't spoil the effect by bleeding into the surrounding skin.

Pressed powder on the lips makes lipstick last longer.

Bite lips to redden them.

To avoid getting lipstick on your teeth, stick your index finger into your mouth, close your lips around it, and pull it out. Any lipstick that was going to go on your teeth should now be on your finger.

Before you go to bed, put vaseline on your lips to keep them soft.

Mix the end of your lipstick in a small pot with some vaseline to make an extra glossy lipstick and not waste the end of the lipstick.

Before you buy a lipstick, try a bit on the back of your hand. The harder it is to wipe off, the longer it will last on your lips.

For a Hollywood smile, put vaseline on the teeth. Why? So your lips aren't sticking to your teeth when you flash your toothy, camera-popping smile.

Toothpastes contain some or all of the following: ammonia, formaldehyde, ethanol, PVP plastics, and sugar. Eeuurgghh. Who needs it?

I make my own natural toothpaste from bicarbonate of soda and peppermint oil.

Get real. I buy the best whitening toothpaste money can buy.

For plaque removal, try fine sea-salt and finish by rubbing the teeth with sage.

I floss my teeth every other day.

Instead of flossing, I sluice out my mouth with lukewarm water after brushing. It's much kinder on my gums.

I used to think braces on teeth were a parental conspiracy to stop their daughters getting kissed. Now I know it's a fashion driven by greedy dentists. Unless you've got teeth like a broken fence or want a job reading the TV news, leave your snappers the way nature intended them.

Dental amalgam contains mercury. When you can, replace old fillings with porcelain, plastic or gold.

Chewing cardamom seeds helps prevent gum disease. They also freshen the breath and aid digestion.

I like a herbal mouthwash made by pouring boiling water onto the flowery tops of meadowsweet. Steep for ten minutes, strain, cool and use.

See off bacteria by rinsing your mouth with a solution of myrrh tincture.

FACE cheeks

To mimic a natural flush, pinch a cheek and see what colour it turns. Then match your blusher to that shade.

You can give yourself better looking cheek bones if you dab a bit of highlighter on the top of your cheek bone, using your fingertips.

If you have forgotten your blusher, use a dab of lipstick on your cheeks and gently blend it in with your fingers.

58

I tone down the glow of my rosy cheeks with a touch of green concealer.

For dry cheeks, apply a mix of one teaspoon of honey, one tablespoon of cream and half a mashed banana. Leave for ten minutes and then wash off.

My grandmother used to recommend rubbing beetroot into the cheeks. Don't ask me why.

To rejuvenate the forehead, apply a little moisturiser or gel to your fingers. Place your middle and third fingers between your eyebrows and glide them upwards and outwards as if smoothing away lines and wrinkles. This is soothing and helps reduce lines.

I carry a pot of Tiger Balm, a soothing ointment that's great for relieving stress. You rub it into your temples and it works miracles on headaches and stress and muscle pains.

A bit of blusher under the chin can help define the chin line.

To firm the chin: start at the edge of the jaw bone on each side, using the thumb and forefinger to pinch the skin gently all the way along the jaw line. Work towards the centre of the chin and back again.

Shoulder length hair is the best way of disguising a receding chin.

A shiny chin? Dab on the powder and the same goes for the nose.

Double chins are to some extent hidden by putting a slightly darker foundation than on the face and running it from the chin into the neck.

Yawn, hold and move your jaw from side to side to work off the beginnings of a double chin.

Chew imaginary pieces of gum for jaw exercise.

To tackle blackheads, steam your face over a bowl of cooling boiled water with added lemon essential oil. Cover your head in a towel over the bowl to trap the steam for five minutes. Then wrap two fingers in tissues, squeeze out the spot and splash your face with cool water.

To cover a spot, apply concealer with a small brush, concentrate on the centre and then feather outwards.

Make sure your concealer is the precise shade of your skin. Otherwise you end up looking like a traffic light with measles.

We've got a juicer and liquidising any of the following has helped my daughter reduce her spots: watercress, carrot, tomato, broccoli, apple, mango, raspberry, apricot and cherry.

If you are going out and find you have a really bad spot, try turning it into a beauty spot with a bit of eyebrow pencil.

Put a dab of toothpaste on spots to draw out the oils.

Spots feed on iodine and those prone to acne should avoid crisps or fish and chips or anything else with lots of salt.

To get rid of a facial spot, dab it with witch hazel during the day and with calamine lotion at night.

I carry a concealer stick to help cover thread veins and the occasional spot.

Spots? Squeezing them is a no-no. Stretch the skin tight by pulling your fingers away from the zit and if it's ready to go, it will go.

If you can't resist squeezing a spot – and few can – go on and squeeeeeeeeeze. It's even more fun than eating chocolate.

Some say that eating chocolate gives you spots.
Rubbish. It's being young that gives you spots, so
enjoy them while you can.

I find that two drops of juniper oil added to a
tablespoon of jojoba or sweet almond oil helps
diminish spots. Apply it with cotton buds.

Another natural spot prevention suggestion is to bathe
the face in a cooled solution of three teaspoons dried
basil boiled in a cup of water.

I put surgical spirit on facial spots.

Dip a cotton bud in tea tree essential oil and dab onto a cold sore, keep going until it dries up.

Rub gold on a cold sore e.g. a ring.

If you get red and blotchy skin in cold weather, put cold compresses on to calm the area.

FACE spots

Only use body lotions and moisturisers when your skin is damp after showering.

For oily skin, use an alcohol-free toner.

Crunchy sea salt and olive oil make a great body scrub.

To heal a scar quickly, break a vitamin E capsule and rub it neat onto the scar.

Bicarbonate of soda makes a good anti-perspirant and avoids the pore-blocking qualities of many shop products.

This combination works for getting a flat stomach. Avoid salty foods and drink at least six large glasses of water a day to avoid fluid retention. Then, from time to time, I do sit-ups starting with twenty-five a day and increasing by five every three days.

For good deportment, pretend you have a board on your head. The old tricks are often the best.

Practice walking by standing in front of a full length mirror and imagine a line from your ears down through your shoulders, hips, knees and ankles. Keep your neck and shoulders relaxed and do a slow, elegant sashay.

Make sure you stand well and keep in mind the classic stuff of shoulders back, stomach in. It sounds dumb but it really will make you look good and feel better.

A little blusher rubbed into the cleavage will make the bust look bigger.

To keep my bust in shape I do this exercise. Kneel on all fours with your arms shoulder width apart. Lower yourself slowly until your nose touches the floor, then come up slowly. Ideally, do this daily about ten times. If you lean further forwards, the exercise is harder but more effective. Basically it makes the pectoral muscles strong and these are the muscles that hold your boobs up.

Wear a bra in bed to keep your boobs firm.

My advice is to take plenty of exercise. Poor skin is often blamed on stress and exercise keeps stress levels down.

The Muriel Spark diet can't fail. She said you simply eat what you normally eat, only half as much. Unlike many diets, this one saves you money by cutting your food bill in half.

Do a little exercise before beginning your day's activities. A fifteen-minute work out will make your circulation better and your face glow.

Quick diets are like quick tans. They can be painful and you tend to lose the advantages as quickly as you gained them.

Lose weight slowly, and then it's more likely to stay off.

As I get older I think more about what I eat and apparently deep coloured foods, particularly fruit and vegetables, are very good for you. So I eat plenty of blackberries, plums, broccoli, spinach and beetroot and, best of all, good, dark chocolate – it does contain iron.

Keep a bowl of fruit on your desk or table.

Drink lashings of water.

If beauty is skin deep, you should know that skin is about 70 per cent water. That's why I try to drink four pints of water every day.

Drink plenty of water or milk before going to a party and eat some fatty food like cheese to line your stomach and slow alcohol absorption. This way you stay upright and look good for longer.

Cut down on the caffeine because it causes dehydration.

Salt helps cause spots.

Drink plenty of healthy juices. Two apples, one banana, one kiwi and 100ml of chilled skimmed milk is good for the skin and tastes delicious.

Eat fresh oranges. The citric acid is good for the complexion.

Sometimes I get bloated with water retention and a drink made up from some of these: cucumber, carrot, parsley, celery, apple, pineapple and cranberry work very well.

Girls shouldn't torture themselves with diets. It's more important to be happy in your skin. In my youth (that was the sixties), the average fashion model weighed no more than 10 per cent less than the average woman. Nowadays, fashion models weigh three-quarters the weight of an average woman. Ask yourself, have average women got 15 per cent fatter or have average models got thinner (and taller)?

CELLULITE

To deal with cellulite, try pummelling the bum and
thighs with the head of a power shower.

My way of dealing with cellulite is exercise and
plenty of water.

A glass of celery juice at bedtime is supposed to help
banish cellulite.

Cellulite? No worries. Get it clear that cellulite is subcutaneous fat that keeps women warm and softens their contours. Until the twentieth century, women and men admired the way flesh dimpled and it took twentieth century advertising to make it seem wrong and something we should get rid of. Germaine Greer is spot on when she says: "Your cellulite is you and will be with you till death or liposuction, which is expensive and extremely painful and sometimes more disfiguring than lumpy fat itself."

To help you tan, take brewer's yeast tablets. This increases the B vitamins in your body that produce the tanning pigment in skin called melanin.

I sometimes use a self-tanning lotion in the winter, especially if I am looking very pale. My skin looks healthier and I feel better.

If you want to give your face a healthy look, use a fake tan and not a foundation. Foundation should always match your skin tone.

If you develop a dark patch when you have done a self-tan rub in toothpaste to counter the effect.

On the principle that beauty is skin deep, you should look after your skin and be in absolutely no doubt that sun is skin's public enemy number one. Rather than thinking of the slimming effects of a tan concentrate on the idea that tanning is the body's ultimately unflattering way of coping with sun damage.

Always, always protect your skin from the sun, especially the face. Use a moisturiser containing a high sun protection factor (SP12-15) on your face, even on cloudy summer days.

Never expose yourself to the dangers of a sun bed. It exposes you to even more ultra-vile ultraviolet than baking yourself in natural sun.

Use sunscreens but realise they have a short life. They lose blocking powers after a couple of years in the bottle and, once applied, are only at their most effective for a maximum of two hours.

Bleaching your hair with sun does more harm than good.

Remember the line about mad dogs and Englishmen . . .

This book's advice for smokers is to go to the doctor when you're ready to quit because most GPs treat smoking as a health issue and will help with a course of Zyban or nicotine gum, or arrange an appointment with a smoking counsellor. Beauty reasons to stop smoking are skin damage, premature wrinkling, dull complexion, smelly breath, stained teeth, squinting, coughing, a gruff voice . . . Enough said.

Speaking as an American, I am amazed at your house prices and at the even more amazing fact that even some really high-priced, high-toned homes get by without a shower. What is it with the Brits that they believe they'll get clean sitting in dirty water?

Rub your body with a loofah or body scrub from your feet upwards before bathing to slough off dry skin and give it a tingly glow.

After a shower, I always put body lotion on to my damp skin before patting dry.

Using a massage mitt after a bath or shower is good
for the circulation and makes you feel firmer.

Soaps are slightly alkaline because this quality helps
loosen dead skin cells and assists in degreasing and
removal of dirt. I prefer soaps that contain glycerine or
olive oil and those made with oatmeal, aloe or
other vegetable bases.

Give yourself a good body scrub. I sprinkle some
sea salt onto a wet flannel and rub, in circular
movements, gently all over my body.

For an instant home sauna, wrap yourself up in a blanket or towel after a warm bath or shower and – if you can bear it – sweat it out for ten minutes. It is important to relax afterwards and drink plenty of water to prevent dehydration and to flush out any remaining toxins.

Add rosemary oil to your bath. This softens the skin and is also very soothing to the nerves.

Add baby oil to bath water to keep the skin soft and moisturised.

You should always apply a moisturiser after a bath because baths actually take moisture out of your skin.

Baths that are too hot open the blood vessels and pores and leave me looking red and mottled.

Step out of a hot bath after a quarter of an hour.

Add some sprigs of fresh rosemary to your hot bath as you run it. It is good for cleansing and smells wonderful.

For soft hands, I rub in baby oil and then put my hands into plastic bags. I tape the bags round the wrists and walk around with my flimsy boxing mittens for fifteen minutes.

Use a good hand cream.

You can make a very good hand scrub by mixing crushed almonds, honey and some lemon juice. Rub this in and you will get rid off dead skin and your hands will feel beautifully moisturised.

Soak rough or chapped hands in a bowl of warm or cold milk for five minutes at night.

I've got a host of wart treatments and most of them make me sound like a witch:

* paint the wart morning and evening with a few drops of thuja or marigold tincture;
* paint the wart morning and evening with the juice from a crushed garlic or a squeezed lemon;
* drink tinctures of Echinacea, burdock, dandelion root or red clover;
* cover onion slices with salt, leave for a few hours and apply juice to skin;
* a drop of juice from a dandelion stalk does the trick;
* visit your doctor.

When you are painting your nails, rest the hand you are painting on a flat surface. Then paint down the centre of the nail and then add a strip either side. This way you do not overload the nails with polish and you get an even finish.

I buy nail capsules, but don't swallow them. Instead, I rub the contents of the capsules straight into the nails.

Sometimes there isn't the time to paint the nails but at least make sure they are cut, filed and buffed to perfection.

Use an acetone-free nail polish remover to stop your nails being stripped of the natural oils that prevent drying out or cracking. Mix vaseline with a few drops of vitamin E oil and rub over your hands. Then put your hands in a plastic bag covered in a towel (so they sweat) and leave for a few minutes.

To stop my nails splitting, I file and reshape them every ten days or so.

Don't paint right to the sides of the nails because it avoids smudging on the skin and makes your nails appear longer.

Keep your nail polish out of direct sunlight.

For flaky nails, slap on some good hand and nail cream.

When filing your nails, go across and in one direction only.

If you haven't time to sit and wait for your nail varnish
to dry then gently apply a drop of baby oil to set
the polish faster.

When you make a bog of painting your nails, use a cotton
bud dipped in remover to tidy the edges.

Give your nails a break from nail varnish every now and then; otherwise they could get weak and discoloured.

Moisturise finger nails in winter as this is when they are more likely to be dry and break.

Keep your hands dry after putting on nail polish because water makes the nail bed expand to stretch the polish and make it prone to chipping.

Dabble nails in lemon juice to restore whiteness after using a dark nail polish.

I broke my nail-biting habit by booking a session with a manicurist a month in advance. The shaming prospect of being revealed as a nail biter was incentive enough to break the habit.

For good nails, make sure you eat:
Vitamin A – fruit and vegetables
B complex – fruit, liver
Vitamin E – wheat germ, egg yolks
Calcium – milk, yoghurt
Magnesium – dried fruits, brown rice
Zinc – seafood and root vegetables

The tops of my arms are dry and get small and knobbly spots so I scour with a body scrub and rub in some moisturiser.

Here's a way to put a bit of definition into the arm muscles. Get a full baked beans tin in each hand; keep shoulders down and arms by the side; keeping the elbows locked, move the arms back as far as possible; don't move the arms forward; don't open the cans of beans.

From *Beauty Adorned* by Elizabeth Ann, 1935: "It is essential in the cult of the beautiful that you have gently rounded tapering arms. Do you possess the sort of arm that tapers from the shoulder into an indent, out again to the elbow, exposes the joint of the elbow, and then finishes, more or less, at a gaunt angle down to your wrist? You are forever going to be arm conscious and at least one third of your enjoyment is going to be marred every time you catch a mirrored or sidelong glance at yourself. Your loveliest gowns will be disappointing if you reveal arms of a different hue from that of your face and throat. Each morning particularly during the warmer months, treat your arms to a brisk patting with your own favoured skin-toning lotion."

My aunt had a tip for what she called prominent elbows. She took the pulp from half a lemon, placed it in the palm of one hand and thrust her elbow into the cupped palm. The prominences (and that's what she called her elbows) thus softened, she then dabbed on a whisper of rouge and the whiteness that made her elbows prominent disappeared altogether.

I apply moisturiser regularly to my elbow. Otherwise the skin cracks.

Always massage the calves after stepping out of a pair of high-heeled shoes.

I do the following regime to firm up my thigh muscles. Stand with feet hip width apart and knees bent. Then squat downwards until your thighs are parallel with the floor. Make sure your back is straight. Slowly return to the starting position. Repeat this. I do three sets of ten with a pause in between, but build up to it.

You can tone up your leg muscles while you have a bath. Grip a sponge between your feet and slowly raise your legs above the water without bending your knees. Keep them straight and hold for a count of five. Repeat several times.

After shaving your legs, apply some moisturiser to make your skin feel extra smooth.

When you have waxed your legs, smooth on a little soya milk as it contains an ingredient that retards hair growth.

Every wet-shave man thinks that shaving foam softens their bristles and this explains why they spend so long in front of the mirror patting their little cheeks. What they don't know is that it is water – and the hotter the better – which softens the hair and the clued-up woman applies the same principle by waiting until the end of the bath before putting her leg razor into action.

When taking off hairs with strip wax, breathe in as you pull the strip off. It eases the pain.

I was getting a scarlet map of broken veins on my thighs and dispelled them with three laser vein removal treatments. If you've got this problem, I'd strongly recommend laser treatment.

About once a week, just before I step into my daily bath, I use a dry brush to rid my legs of any dry skin.

If your shins are dry and flaky mix some oatmeal with a rich moisturiser, smooth over legs and then rinse off.

If your feet are tired after a long day at work, fill a bowl with warm water, drop in a few soluble aspirin tablets and dunk the feet. The acid in the aspirins will soften callouses and hard skin.

For a quick foot massage, put marbles in the bottom of a bowl of warm water and roll your feet around. Then rub the dead skin away with a pumice stone or stiff brush.

Don't cut your nails too short or too rounded as this can cause in-growing nails.

Carry a foot spray to lighten up your feet during the day.
Very refreshing.

Soak your feet in warm water and add a few drops of the
essential oil of your choice. I use camomile to soften,
lavender for healing and peppermint for cooling.

Put conditioning cream [or vaseline] on your feet last
thing at night, then put some socks on. By morning
the cream will have penetrated the driest layers
and your feet will be really soft.

Jiggle and circle ankles to keep them slim.

I never shop for clothes without a friend. A second opinion – even if it's that of your best enemy – is vital and stops you being pressurised by sales people.

Get measured whenever you buy a new bra, because you do not stay the same size forever.

Prepare yourself for shopping. For example, wear the right kind of bra, shoes and tights for the party dress you're going to buy. Ankle socks won't let you judge the effect.

For cheaper items, dark colours are best. Things that are lightly coloured have to be better cut and well stitched to look good.

Dress well when you buy clothes. That way the assistants won't be so intimidating and you won't feel you're trying to buy a way of turning an ugly duckling into a swan.

When shopping, go with a mission. Write a list and stick to your plan. That's a rule for life, isn't it? Well rule number two is to break rule number one in the event of an irresistible sale item or anything else that suddenly seems interesting.

When I go shopping I make sure I have comfortable shoes for all that walking and I also wear clothes I can tear off quickly and easily in the changing room.

I take a bottle of water and an apple with me when I go shopping. Without refreshments, I get headachy and come back home empty handed.

I think the best wardrobe is classic clothes in plain colours; then you can add colour by buying cheap seasonal items.

Have a full-length mirror. It's impossible to get dressed
properly without one.

If wearing a top without a bra, put plasters on your
nipples. When it gets cold it won't look as
if you're smuggling peanuts.

If you like to wear bras with tops but the straps are going to
show attach things to the straps. Depending on time and
place you could stick on diamante or sew on beads or little
embroidered flowers.

Never wear horizontal stripes if you are large.

If wearing a vee neck, low-top dress use double-sided tape to hold the fabric to the breast to prevent gaping.

With a low-cut top, you can highlight the collar bones with a bit of bronzing powder or glitter, depending on the time of day.

Use toupee tape to hold clothes in place if you are wearing a low-cut dress.

If you need to fix your hem in an emergency you can use double-sided sellotape.

Wear a G-string to get rid of the visible panty line.

If wearing tight trousers and you don't want a VPL and you don't like thongs then wear little hot pants, they are low cut and come under the buttocks.

If you've got very long legs, don't wear pinstripes or you will look like a clown. But for somebody short, pinstripes are perfect.

Rub a bar of soap into laddered tights. It will do while you're out.

To deter moths, wrap woollen garments in newspaper before you store them over the summer.

To get the creases out of your clothes, hang them up in the bathroom when you take a shower.

Hang dark coloured skirts and blouses inside out. This way the dust specks that gather do not show.

Fold clothes crosswise not lengthwise, because the folds drop out more quickly.

Roll synthetic fabrics instead of folding them.
That way, they crease less.

If you have a really long dress to store, sew loops at waist
level inside. Turn the bodice part over the skirt and put on
the hanger from the loops. This will keep the hem from
crumpling and getting dusty.

Store and hang your clothes in colour coordinations. It's an
easy way to keep smart.

Put coats and jackets on hangers so you don't get vee-shaped
hook marks, or distort the fabric.

Use decent wooden coat hangers.

Put one item per coat hanger.

To stop clothes from sliding off hangers stick a bit of foam plastic around the shoulder of the hanger.

Wire coat hangers distort clothes. Unravel them to poke down blocked drains. That's all they're good for.

When a zip sticks, try spraying it with silicone furniture polish.

Lightweight jumpers can be hung up to dry without losing their shape by threading a pair of tights through the sleeves and attaching to the clothes line.

If you stain silk clothes, a spray cleaner may just seal in the stain or make a mark of its own. Trust the experts and go to a dry cleaners.

To remove chewing gum from clothes, put in the freezer and chip off the gum when it has frozen.

Before washing a really precious wool sweater, trace its outline onto some stout card. Then you can stretch it back to its right size and shape after washing.

Your garment is clean, dry – but creased. To flatten it, put it in the fridge for ten minutes.

If your black clothes are looking a bit grey, try soaking them in a bowl of warm water with half a cup of vinegar added to it. The greyness may be just a build-up of washing powder.

If you've got shoe polish stains on your socks, put a bit of methylated spirit on the stain before washing.

To make your tights last longer rinse them in warm water, wring out gently, then put them in a plastic bag and secure. Leave them in the freezer and thaw out next day.

If you get mud anywhere on your clothes, always let it dry before you brush it, otherwise you just spread the mud.

To get rid of creases, hang clothes in a steamy bathroom.

To get rid of grease spots iron fabric over a piece of brown paper.

Be careful of stain removers on clothes. Many contain benzene, sulphamic acid and toluene and these ingredients can give you spots.

When you spill red wine on your clothes, sprinkle the stain thickly with salt and brush it out later after it has dried.

To clean trainers, put them in a pillowcase so they don't ruin the washing machine and put the machine on its coolest setting so it doesn't ruin the trainers. Don't dry them by a radiator and do stuff the toes when they are drying to keep the shape. Wash the laces separately and iron them or buy new ones.

If your socks are likely to be seen, make sure they are either attractive or fun. I like fishnet socks.

If you have shoes or boots with pointy toes, keep a ball of cotton wool in the tip of the toe to protect from dents. Leave in when wearing.

When wearing a new pair of shoes, always carry plasters.
They should sell plasters and chocs in the loos at clubs.
More girls come in complaining of painful feet and needing
a sugar hit than needing sanitary towels or condoms.

If your boots and shoes are looking tired go to a good
menders and have them re-soled, re-heeled and polished.
They will look like new and last much longer.

Avoid wearing knee-high boots if you are short.
Instead wear calf-length boots because they make
your legs look longer.

If you like wearing high heels, have at least two pairs of shoes with a different height of heel. This varies the strain your calf muscles will take and could prevent swelling.

Buy the best shoes and boots that you can and look after them.

If you want to be able to wear a pair of trousers with both trainers and heels put velcro on the hem. Velcro up for trainers, peel down for heels.

For strappy shoes, don't forget to put a bit of tan on the feet and ankles.

If shoes are uncomfortable when you try them on, don't buy them. They rarely get more comfortable with wearing.

Leather shrinks in the heat, so remember not to store your shoes under a radiator.

The thinner the heel the longer the leg looks.

For the white, salty lines on your shoes from rain or snow wipe with a little white vinegar.

If you have chunky ankles, don't wear shoes with straps.

ACCESSORIES

Wear larger earrings when your hair is short or drawn up
and off your face.

Patent leather shoes and handbags will stay supple if you
occasionally rub them with olive oil.

If you are wearing white or cream clothes, use
pale accessories as well.

Carry a small handbag and don't stuff it. It forces you
to be ruthless about what you carry with you and stops you
looking like a bag lady.

Were I to be able to turn the clock back to 1977, I'd be a
punk and carry a kettle for a handbag

Ever since I got married, I haven't lost a single glove.

119

To soften dry skin rub a teaspoonful of vegetable oil into any dry patches before going to bed.

Never go to sleep with your makeup on.

To prevent my skin from drying out, I swear by a night cream. I put it on half an hour before bed by blotting my face with a tissue.

I never go to bed without my teddy.

I have a routine to avoid tossing and turning all night.
Ten minutes before retiring I take four drops of the
original Bach's Rescue Remedy. I take my make-up
off, put my jim-jams and hand cream on, bang my
head on the pillow three times and uncoil every
part of my body. The routine works even better
with two glasses of red wine.

Sleep. Beauty. The two words go together so try reading
SLEEP: 365 ways to drop off.

YOUR TIPS

GETTING GOING

HAIR care

HAIR brushing

HAIR washing/conditioning

HAIR dandruff

EYE care

EYEbrows

EYElashes

· EYElids

MAKEUP

FACE washing

FACE exfoliating

FACE toning

FACE the shape

FACE the lips

FACE the teeth

FACE the cheeks

FACE the forehead

FACE the chin

SPOTS AND COLD SORES

THE BODY

DIETS AND CELLULITE

TANNING for and against

SMOKING

YOUR TIPS

125

BATHS

HANDS

NAILS

ARMS

ELBOWS

LEGS

FEET

CLOTHES buying

CLOTHES wearing

CLOTHES storing

CLOTHES washing

FOOTWEAR

ACCESSORIES

GOING TO BED